Press RESET for Longevity

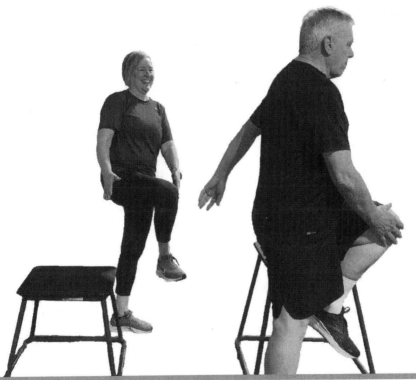

original strength

original strength

Pressing RESET for Longevity

Copyright © 2023 Original Strength Systems, LLC

ALL RIGHTS RESERVED.

All rights reserved solely by the copyright holder. The copyright holder guarantees all contents are original and do not infringe upon the legal rights of any other person or work. No part of this book may be reproduced or transmitted in any form or by any means, electronic or mechanical, including photocopying, recording or by any information storage and retrieval system, without the permission of the copyright holder or the publisher.

Published by OS Press - Fuquay-Varina, NC

Contributor: Suzie Gullett Strength and Movement Specialist

ISBN:
Paperback: 979-8-9865860-5-2

Medical Disclaimer

This booklet is not here to treat, diagnose, or prescribe for any physical condition. It's important to note that this is simply a guide for those looking for healthy, happy aging. This does not trump the medical advice from your doctor or a professional. If at any time you experience pain when following this guide, STOP. DON'T MOVE INTO PAIN – pain changes how you move. A regression may be required. We are here to show how the human body was designed to move. In the process of moving correctly, good things can happen. However, it would also be advised to seek advice from a medical professional if you are having pain.

Having said that, here is how Original Strength (OS) -Original Strength is a lot to type so let's just go with OS, OK? - helps you live life better and stronger.

Pressing RESET for Longevity

Pressing RESET is the Original Strength term for a full body reset. Not a clearing or an erasing, but a way to start with a new baseline and, from there, progress to your best.

Longevity is the ability to live within ideal conditions as long as you can or as long as you are able. In other words, your life experiences, what you have accomplished, what you know, and what you have become set a course for your longevity.

Using Original Strength, you can live and move in an abundant life because of your design - one that provides an extraordinary life of longevity. We know that each movement you have was designed for you so that you can live and move well your entire life.

Often as we age, we collect life experiences that may deter us from truly living to the best of our ability. Usually, one's relationship with their parents, who either dealt with their own injuries or failed to encourage physical activity, has set a poor example. Or perhaps you have bought into the idea that as you get older, you should feel your age and accept the limits that come with it. Many even believe that we have a prime, and after passing that prime we lose the ability to live well and move well.

The Original Strength model tells us to never move into pain, breathe through our nose, develop our balance through eye and head movements, find our best movement through simple gait patterns, and believe the fact that our design is perfect. It's important to know that you were designed to live well your whole life. And most importantly, no matter how well you move now, you can hit that reset button and move and live even better.

In this book, you will see how you can:

- Connect to your best movement
- Learn to feel better
- Increase your strength without a gym and its expensive equipment

And all in as little as 1-10 minutes a day.

Here are a few examples of people who have made long-lasting changes in their movement. I will also introduce you to my personal inspiration to move well my entire life.

Wilma

Born 1908 *(Or should we say "Lived to be 99")*

My grandmother lived a life that more closely matched how we are designed to move. Until the day she died at 99, she never stopped baking bread, hanging her laundry out to dry, and walking around San Diego because she never learned to or saw the need to drive a car. She read her bible from sunup to sundown. She was amazing. She went home to the Lord at age 99 without medication, significant surgeries, or illnesses. She is my main inspiration - showing me that movement and a good attitude is what longevity is all about.

Elaine

Born 1936 *(Or should we say "86 Years Old")*

A single mother raising a son and knew the importance of taking care of herself. Not just for the example to her son but because she saw the slow decline of her parents, who slowly decreased their movement and activity. She saw her parents break their hips, have chronic heart issues, and reduce their activity levels due to diabetes. She wanted something different for her life. She chooses every day to Press RESET in her movement. She has learned how to breathe and release stress and how to move in ways that allow her to live and feel better.

Jeff

Born 1956 *(Or should we say "66 Years Old")*

Technically a senior, Jeff lives his best life every day. He has made it a point to learn to ride long distances and join and lead 100-mile bike rides for Team in Training. Jeff was diagnosed with stage 4 prostate cancer and knew that to maintain the strength he needed for the rigorous chemotherapy and radiation treatments, he would have to continue to move every day. He learned to use the three pillars of Pressing RESET: diaphragmatic breathing, eye movements (head control) and crossing the midline of his body daily. Jeff credits Pressing RESET with helping his recovery from surgery, maintaining strength and mobility, and keeping his balance. Jeff is off medications and continues to improve in all areas of movement and longevity.

These are a few examples of how movement can change you, strengthen you and maintain your ability to live and move well your entire life.

Pressing RESET

RESET #1

Pressing RESET Every Day

Every day, probably without knowing it, you do the three things which are the basis of all movement. Using one of the three with the proper intent and focus can help your body move better and increase your longevity. But putting all three together with intention can be a game-changer to how you feel, move and live.

Three Pillars of Human Movement

- **Diaphragmatic Breathing**
- **Eye Movements and Head Movements**
- **Crossing the Midline of Your Body, Otherwise Known as Walking**

With any of the movements you're going to do, a crucial part of Original Strength is that you never move into pain. If you quickly get into pain when doing any of these movements, be careful to move slowly and allow the body to do less to avoid pain. Pain is the body's way of requesting a change in your actions.

Before we begin practicing some RESET methods, it is important to see where your body is today regarding movement. Let's start with what we call a "baseline check-in." A baseline check-in, or movement check, is a simple, repeatable body movement. Your baseline can be turning your head, raising your arms overhead, reaching down and touching your toes, or even squatting. After each RESET, you can recheck your baseline to see if it feels the same as when you tested, better than when you first tested, or perhaps you feel the best you have in a relatively long time.

So let's pick a baseline movement to check and recheck through the first RESETS. Turn your head gently right and left. Do you feel clicking, cracking or popping? How far can you turn your head? Is it the same on both sides? Your baseline can be either or both quantitative or qualitative.

Before we start with our first RESET, let's use turning our heads as our baseline check. Do that now. Do not move into pain.

Movement 1

DIAPHRAGMATIC BREATHING/NASAL BREATHING

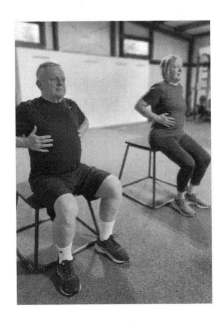

Our design is to breathe through our noses and deep into our lungs. Diaphragmatic breathing, or what some call "belly breathing," is critical for balanced health, well-being and movement. It notably assists with stress relief, digestion, hormone production and bladder control.

Try This

- Gently turn your head right and left. Sit tall, and place your hands on your belly at the bottom of your ribcage. Place your tongue on the roof of your mouth like when you swallow. Begin to breathe through your nose.

Breathe slowly and deeply expand the belly as you inhale for ten slow breaths.

- Now, recheck your head turn. Does it feel or sound different? Is it less crunchy (e.g., clicking, cracking, popping)? Can you turn even a little further? Do you feel more relaxed?

That is the beauty of diaphragmatic breathing.

Movement 2

EYE MOVEMENTS

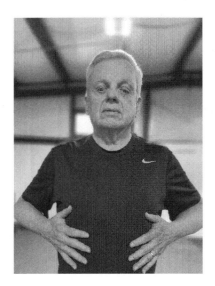
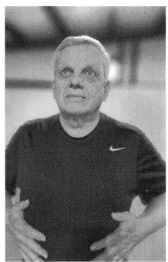

Moving multi-directionally is the natural design for our eyes. However, due to glasses, surgeries, computer use, etc., we limit the range of motion of our eyes. Yes, just like your arms or legs, your eyes are attached to muscles that get weak and tired and lose their range of motion.

HEAD TURNS

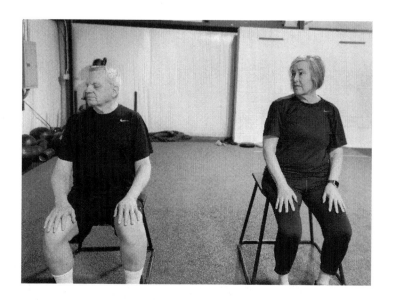

Try This

- Look forward with your eyes open. Keep your tongue on the roof of your mouth. Focus on breathing into your belly. By moving your eyes, look up and down, repeating ten times. Again, moving only your eyes, look left to right ten times.
- Alternatively, with each eye movement, you can move your eyes in one direction entirely, then move your head to where you're looking. Let your eyes move first, then let your head follow.
- Now, recheck your head turn. Is it less crunchy? Can you turn even a little further? Is there any pain?

Movement 3

CROSSING THE MIDLINE - "CROSS CRAWLING"

By design, as a baby we go through many movements to ultimately walk. When we walk, our arms move in opposition to each other, which rotates the midline of our body. Crossing our midline helps our brain to reconnect our body's natural movement patterns. Even if our walking is limited, there are modified ways to practice this movement.

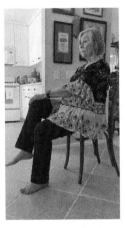 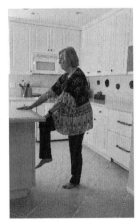 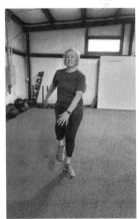

Seated *Supported* *Standing*

All of these movements can be practiced individually or combined to increase their effectiveness.

Try This

- Sitting up in a chair, position yourself so you are not resting against the backrest. With your eyes open, keep your tongue on the roof of your mouth, breathe through your nose into your belly, touch your right hand to your left knee, and alternate your left hand to your right knee for about ten taps on each side.
- Now, recheck your head turn. Is it less crunchy? Can you turn even a little further? Any pain?
- These pillars of human movement are the basis of all of our movement. We can increase the range of our movement, modify how we move, or even combine movements to increase, decrease or change the challenge of any movement.

RESET #2

Live Better, Not Just Longer

Longevity is more than just lifespan, it is connected to how we move in that life.

Remember, longevity is how well we live within the conditions in which we live. We often don't perceive our situation as ideal, but we can change that. We are not in a fixed system of evolving. We can grow, change, move and feel better at any age. You were designed to live well your entire life. Let's learn to reset our thinking and live better.

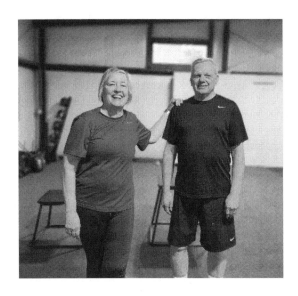

For many, the fear of falling is as bad - or even worse - than the fear of public speaking. It may be that we merely think we are clumsy or not coordinated, but falling has a lot to do with our breathing and eyes.

Our eyes and our breathing are crucial in any movement we do. If you are not breathing well, your body is restraining your movement. It is your brain's job to keep you safe. We often trick our body into feeling unsafe - we don't always realize we are holding our breath or staring. Our breath needs to move freely and our eyes need to move around to see everything. If your eyes are fixed in one position, your body will not always know where to turn and you may become unsteady or even fall. Reconnecting to better breathing and eye movements are a means to regain a better balance and teach our body that it is safe to move.

> "Remember, longevity is how well we live within the conditions in which we live"

Practicing breathing and eye movements while seated is a great way to teach your body how to move well in a calm environment.

Let's try a couple of breathing exercises. You can do these while standing at a counter or behind a steady chair.

Try This

1. Breathing - 1 minute

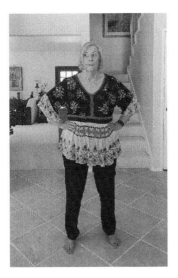

2. Head nods and turns - 1 minute

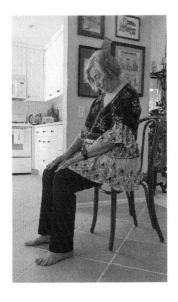

3. Cross Crawls - 1 minute

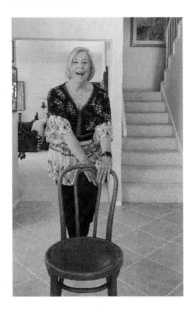

After you feel confident in the three basic RESETS we've discussed, you might be ready to add some extra RESETS to help your body begin to become more resilient and add to your longevity.

Remember we were designed to move well our entire life.

Elaine and Jeff, whom we mentioned above, both have a mindset for movement. However, both of them had some serious, potentially game-changing life situations. They learned from their experiences that it does feel good to feel good. Adding movements is how you become more comfortable through each RESET.

As you progress in using the Original Strength RESETS you will begin to feel your body moving better and responding to stimuli and stresses better which will help you to develop your longevity. As you use the resets you will become more confident in your movement. You will notice that you are able to make movements that were once causing you stress more relaxing. You will especially see - if you start small - that you will be able to move with a greater range of motion and move longer and with more strength and confidence. Remember you were designed for movement and then add these movements to really make your body feel better and more able.

There are some pictures of more challenging RESETS you can move into, such as Knees Rocking, Circles and Bird Dog. Always start slow and progress from where you are. Your body will tell you or give you permission with better access to movement when it is ready.

Movement 1

KNEES ROCKING

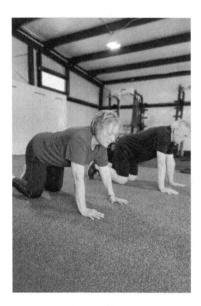
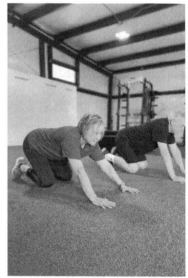

Movement 2

CIRCLES

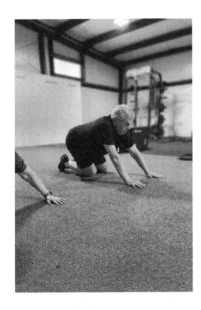 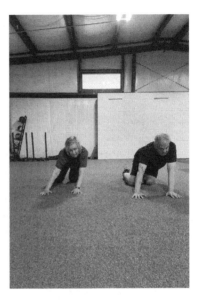

Movement 3

BIRD DOG

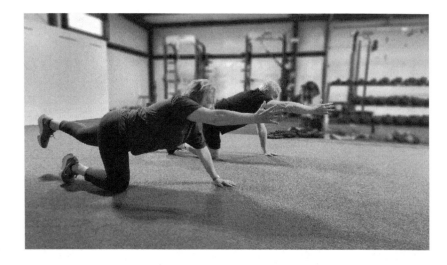

RESET #3

Pressing RESET Anywhere

A common fear for many is the fear of falling. Maybe a friend or parent has fallen and it has reduced your confidence in moving. We find that instead of taking the chances of falling, many choose to not take any chances at all, and they stop moving altogether. Remember movement is a relationship between you and your body.

Original Strength helps you press the reset button on how you are thinking and gives you the tools to become more balanced. We have a reflexive or righting mechanism built into us that we can keep sharp and fine tune if we keep moving and working on controlling our head. When we were a baby it was all about getting our head steady. Believe it or not, as we grow up it's no different. Your body follows your head, which follows your eyes.

You have so many opportunities and options to move your body when you take into account where you are starting from today, where you can progress to, and listening to what is best for you. We like to remind people to "start where you are, use what you have, and do what you can".

Standing Pressing RESET for Better Balance

A 3-minute daily practice to increase your balance

- 1-minute diaphragmatic breathing
- 1-minute eye movements and head movements
- 1-minute rotating the body

Start with a quick assessment standing next to a chair or by a counter. Pick up one foot and balance. Count how long you can balance while standing on each foot. Don't forget to reassess yourself after you are done.

START STANDING

(If you want to use a stable chair or stand close to the counter that is a great option.)

Movement 1

BREATHING

First minute

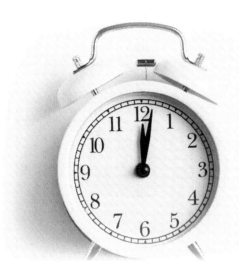

- Set a kitchen timer for one minute, or do this 10 times
- Breathe into your belly or diaphragmatically

Movement 2

EYE MOVEMENTS AND HEAD MOVEMENTS

Second minute

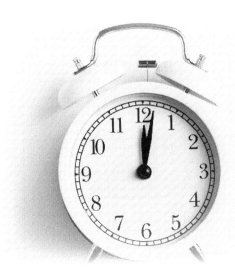

- Begin by looking up and down, moving only your eyes for about five times.
- Slowly add a nodding with your head as if to say "yes."
- Then follow move your eyes left and right.
- Slowly add a turn of your head as if to say" No."

Movement 3

ROTATE AROUND THE MIDLINE OF THE BODY

Third minute

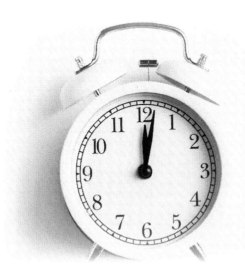

Begin to turn, but do it in this sequence:

1. Eyes look
2. Head follows
3. Body follows (shoulders, ribs, hips, foot)

Start small and continue to rotate as much as is comfortable for you. Try to return to the starting position in the same manner but reverse (foot, hips, ribs, shoulder, head) and repeat to the other side.

You have decided to move better and as your body was designed with your own set of experiences. You may have had an injury in your past to your head or neck which can make movement difficult. Remember, start where you are. Try to always do a baseline move before you begin a new session, and progress as your body is ready.

Most OS RESETS can be done seated, standing supported or unsupported. Even if you are doing the RESETS while seated you can still check your balance before and after.

The body is amazing and can do great things.

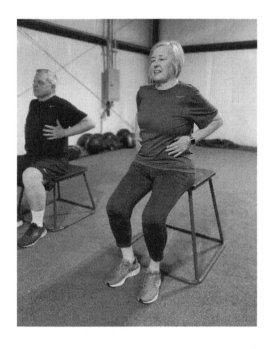

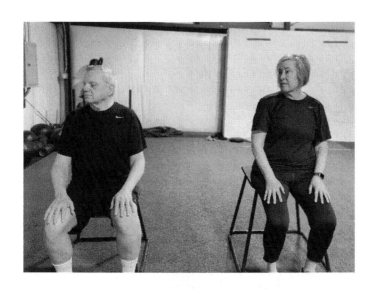

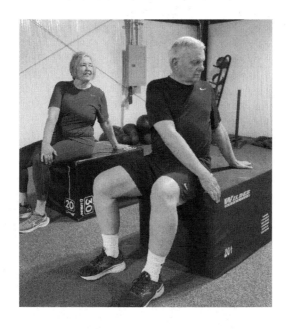

RESET 4

Pressing RESET for Better Movement

We were designed to move in so many ways. We can bend and lift and turn. We also can balance and stabilize ourselves while turning and reaching to put something away on a low shelf or even up high in a closet.

Our movement can be reset so our reflexive ability to stay stable helps us. Our reflexive strength and balance is the internal part of us that supports and protects us in all of our movements even when we are not thinking about it. Think about when you stumble as you are walking and your body automatically catches itself so you don't fall. That is the reflexive strength that you have. We want to use our RESETS to build up our reflexive strength.

Let's start to Press RESET to build up movements.

Rocking, Rolling, and Cross Crawling

Movement 1

ROCKING

Rocking helps to strengthen your whole body. When you were still ambling around on all fours as a baby, rocking was preparation for walking. Rocking developed and will continue to develop strength in your joints - toes, ankles, knees, hips, the spine, wrist, shoulders and neck. As we begin to walk, wear shoes, learn to compensate for sitting for long hours and forget to take walks, our body's joints become stiffer. The old adage "use it or lose it" comes into play here.

Except, we don't lose our movements! We can still sort of do what we need to. We can walk, get out of a chair and take part in sports but now our joints have become stiff, tired and sore. We often blame aging. Even the doctor may say, "Well, you are getting older," and chalk up your symptoms to old age. Remember movement is part of our design. We were not meant to wear out before we need to. So even if you feel like you have joints that are older than your age, know that you should start where you are, progress as you need to. Be steady and consistent in your movements and you will start to move and feel better than you do now!

This is one of the big principles of Original Strength. *Start where you are today.* Not back on the floor as a 6-month-old. Not back in high school when you were on that team. Not even where you were yesterday. Each day is an opportunity to move better, to feel better and in turn, live better. Start where you are. Start today and meet yourself where you are at.

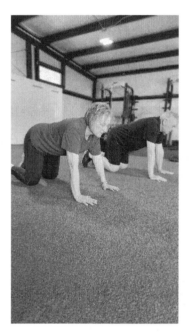 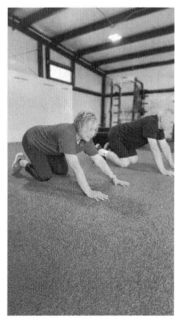

Movement 2

ROLLING

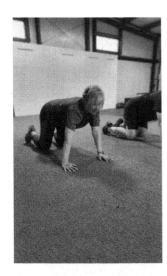
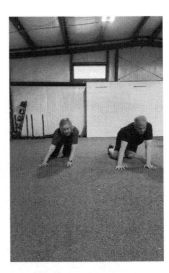
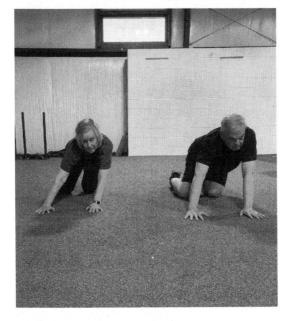

Movement 3

CROSS-CRAWLING OR BIRD DOG

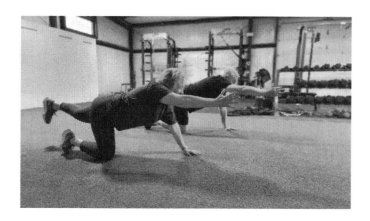

CROSS CRAWLS

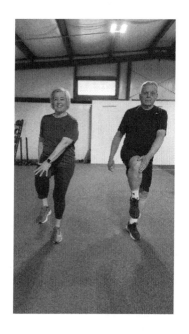

Some RESETS to get you started:

Set up two chairs approximately 3 feet apart
Start in one chair with
1-minute breathing
1-minute head nods and head turns
1 min on seated cross crawls
Stand up and walk in a figure 8 pattern around the chair until you return to your first chair.

Variations
Do 4-6 laps
Sit down in each seat you come to

Or

Walk backward around the chair

Or

Do a cross crawl as you walk around the chairs

Try This

- Stand next to a kitchen counter or even a lower stable surface
- Hands-on the counter
- Breathe 1 minute, while breathing, add eye movements and head movements and then add cross crawls to both. Go slow and only pick up the pace if you can

continue to breathe with your mouth closed with your tongue at the roof of your mouth.

Try This

- Using a kitchen counter or stable surface, even a chair seat
- Stand at counter
- Begin with breathing followed by eye and head movements
- Add a rocking movement
- Shift hips back toward heels and straighten out arms shift back to the counter
- Add opposition movement
- Bird dog (pictured on page X)
- Lift right arm and left leg and then repeat with the left arm and right leg
- Cross Crawl
- Stand tall touch right hand to left knee and left hand to right knee

More Tips as you RESET

- Don't limit yourself.
- Don't let anyone else limit you.
- Let your movement progress.
- Be kind to yourself, you have had many experiences.

- Find a friend to Press RESET with. Every day is a new day. Start where you are that day. Growth, change and progress will happen.
- Press RESET outside.
- Press RESET barefoot.
- Press RESET while waiting in line.
- Combine different RESETS - like standing and sitting or sitting on the floor and standing.
- Press RESET on the carpet or the tile or your wood floor. The body likes to move in different ways.
- Set small goals and give yourself a small reward when you reach a goal.

Your
DESIGN

Longevity Will Find You

Allow yourself to move more, and live well. Pressing RESET for longevity will help you live better, and longer while better. Learn to know the feeling of feeling good. As Tim Anderson, the founder of Original Strength, likes to say, "It feels good to feel good".

I hope you let yourself return to great movement. Move better and live better

Even if you did one minute of diaphragmatic breathing each day you would begin to notice the benefits of better movement.

- Standing taller
- More mentally connected
- Release of tension in hips knees and neck

If you want to learn more about Original Strength log on to Youtube and check out some of the "Movement Snax"

The Movement Snax are 3-5 minute videos showing you ways you can move differently, move better and develop longevity in all things.

Want to learn more?

This booklet was designed to give a brief overview of the Original Strength System and how it can help you Press RESET on how you move to help your longevity.

We put it together because we know it can help everyone and anyone. If you do nothing more than what is in this booklet, you will notice many changes in how your mind and body begin to feel and react to various situations.

Original Strength is a human movement education company with a mission to bring the hope and strength of movement to everybody in the world. Based on the human developmental sequence and the human body's design, the Original Strength System teaches movements that help RESET an individual's neuromuscular system, allowing them to enjoy improved physical movement and physiological function.

We conduct courses, training, and certifying coaches and instructors. We also develop educational materials for PE teachers, physical therapy students, medical professionals, fitness/health/wellness instructors, sports conditioning professionals, and individuals/groups working with vestibular and neuromuscular functionality.

Some RESETS to get you started: If you want to know more about Pressing RESET and regaining your original strength, visit originalstrength.net. There you will find a variety of books, hundreds of free video tutorials (**OS Movement Snax**), and a complete listing of our courses and OS Certified Professionals near you.

You may want to consider finding an OS Certified Professional. These professionals will conduct an Original Strength Screen and Assessment (OSSA), which is the quickest and easiest way to identify areas your movement system needs to go from good to best. The OSSA allows a pro to pinpoint the best place for you to start Pressing RESET and restoring your Original Strength.

We encourage you to reach out to the OS team with any questions you may have. ***Please keep us updated with your progress; we really want to know how you are doing - progress@OriginalStrength.net.*** Press RESET now and live life better & stronger because you were awesomely and wonderfully made to accomplish amazing things.

Press RESET now and live life better because you were awesomely and wonderfully made to accomplish amazing things.

For more information:

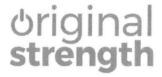

Original Strength Systems, LLC
OriginalStrength.net

PressingRESETfor@Originalstrength.net

"... I am fearfully and wonderfully made..."
Psalm 139:14

Made in the USA
Columbia, SC
17 May 2025